Donald k. Cilley

THE CORNEAL BLINDNESS IMPLANT

How the implant of a pig protein recapture a human vision

Copyright © 2022 by Donald k. Cilley

All rights reserved. No part of this publication may be reproduced, stored or transmitted in any form or by any means, electronic, mechanical, photocopying, recording, scanning, or otherwise without written permission from the publisher. It is illegal to copy this book, post it to a website, or distribute it by any other means without permission.

First edition

This book was professionally typeset on Reedsy
Find out more at reedsy.com

Contents

INTRODUCTION

Ocular damage is prevalent; in the United States, it affects an estimated 24 million people.

.[1]

The degree of eye injuries varies, ranging from a minor corneal scratch (corneal abrasion) to a split in the exterior structure (globe rupture). One instance of a globe rupture in the eye is a laceration of the cornea. A corneal laceration was seen in 20.7% of the 890 eye injuries that were examined from 2001 to 2011 in Iraq and Afghanistan.

[2]

Corneal lacerations can range from a straightforward linear pattern to a complicated stellate formation, are different in size and shape, and can be partial or full thickness. To lower the danger of infection, lessen tissue necrosis, and minimize patient suffering, all lacerations need to be repaired very away. The usual time frame for a repair recommendation is 24 hours.

[3]Cerebral lacerations are frequently repaired with sutures; however, lacerations smaller than 2 mm can be stitched together using tissue adhesives or contact lenses.

Any repair must achieve a watertight closure, return to normal anatomy, and minimize astigmatism and corneal scarring after surgery. [4]

THE CORNEAL

Cornea.

The transparent, dome-shaped cornea is a part of the front of the eye.

Its optical power is around forty-three diopters, however, the typical range is rather broad. There is no blood supply to it.

A thin tear film that provides an exceptionally smooth optical surface covers the cornea.

The collagen fibers' neat arrangement is related to the cornea's transparency. It contains no water. The endothelial cells in the cornea pump the water out of it, keeping it "dry." Corneal edema can be brought on by any condition that affects the corneal endothelium. The tissue will become less translucent as a result, harming its optical properties.

The target of the most popular refractive procedures, like LASIK, is the cornea.

It is also a reasonably simple organ to transplant. After a corneal graft, long-term systemic immunosuppression is not required.

MENDING OF CORNEAL TEAR

Ocular trauma frequently results in corneal lacerations. To lower the danger of infection, ease patient suffering, and prevent future eye injury, repair should take place within 24 hours. A watertight closure, the return of normal anatomy, and the avoidance of severe astigmatism or scarring are the objectives of the repair.

Can a ripped cornea be fixed?

The cornea may still quickly heal itself even in the presence of disease or injury. But occasionally, as with a serious corneal injury, the damage is too extensive for the cornea to recover on its own.

Steps you can take right away if you have a corneal abrasion

Clean water or a saline solution should be used to rinse your eye. Use a tiny, clean drinking glass with the rim resting on the bone at the base of your eye socket or an eyecup.

Blink numerous times.

Overlap the upper and lower eyelids.

CORNEAL PPMD

Cornea Category(ies): Posterior Polymorphous Corneal Dystrophy (PPMD)

A rare, bilateral, inherited corneal dystrophy known as posterior polymorphous corneal dystrophy (PPMD, PPCD) is caused by an autosomal dominant gene. Rarely will corneal edema or raised intraocular pressure result from the corneal abnormalities in PPMD, which is located at the level of Descemet's membrane and endothelium. Band lesions, diffuse deep stromal opacities, and endothelial vesicle-like lesions are the three primary patterns in which PPMD may manifest.

Vesicle-like lesions in PPMD are seen in

Figure 1.

The distinctive lesions of PPMD are vesicle-like lesions at the level of Descemet's membrane and endothelium. They typically form in lines or groups and have the appearance of translucent cystic lesions encircled by gray haloes. The illustrations below show how these lesions typically appear under direct illumination, retro illumination, and specular microscopy.

Figure 2: PPMD, CRA band lesions

Band lesions, often known as "snail tracks," are typically horizontal lesions at the level of the posterior cornea with parallel, scalloped, non-tapering borders. Examples of these lesions in 2 different patients are shown below.F

Figure3: PPMD, CRA diffuse posterior stromal opacities

Diffuse, gray-white opacities at the level of Descemet's membrane may be a PPMD symptom. The area around the lesions may have a thick stromal haze. The two patients with these lesions are seen in the slit lamp images below.

Confocal microscopy of the PPMD-affected endothelium is shown in

Figure 4.The endothelium in PPMD exhibits epithelial-like cells under confocal imaging. Flat and hexagonal endothelial cells are typical.

CORNEAL REFLEX

The corneal reflex, often referred to as the blink reflex or eyelid reflex, is an uncontrollable blinking of the eyelids that is brought on by stimulation of the cornea, though it can also be brought on by any other peripheral stimuli. There should be a direct and unanimous response to stimulation. The reflex happens quickly, at a pace of 0.1 seconds.

How to perform corneal reflex

When the cornea is irritated by being touched with a sterile cotton applicator, the corneal reflex is assessed by the closure of the eyelids. The trigeminal nerve sends afferent impulses, whereas the facial nerve sends efferent motor impulses.

corneal reflex normally

The corneal reflex, sometimes referred to as the blink reflex or the eyelid reflex, is an uncontrollable blinking of the eyelids that is brought on by stimulation of the cornea (such as by touching or by a foreign body), though it can also be brought on by any peripheral input.

inadequate corneal reflex

When something touches your eye, this response makes you blink in order to shield the surface of your eye from harm.

1. **Testing of the corneal reflex** is frequently included in a neurological evaluation. You may have a nerve, brain, or ocular illness if this reaction is weakened and your eye does not blink when touched.

Causes of the eye's reflex action

The pupils of both eyes constrict when a light is flashed close to one of them. The reaction is sent to the pupillary musculature by autonomic nerves that supply the eye after the brain receives impulses from the optic nerve as the stimuli. The lacrimal reflex is another reflex that affects the eye.

CORNEAL MOLDING

Orthokeratology is the more common name for corneal molding (CM). It involves changing the cornea's curvature as you sleep using fancy hard gas permeable contact lenses called corneal molds. When the patient removes the lens after awakening, they are able to see clearly all day WITHOUT ANYTHING IN THEIR EYES.

It is suitable for persons of all ages, including those who need bifocals or have myopia, hyperopia, astigmatism, or both (presbyopia). For the younger patient who experiences ongoing vision deterioration (stronger glasses every year...), a key additional benefit is that this molding process ceases, which considerably slows that trend. One of the most common queries from parents is, "How can I prevent my child's eyes from getting worse every year?" This alone provides the answer.

How to prevent your eyes from growing worse

Put the corneal molds in your eyes before going to bed, sleep with them in, remove them when you wake up, and see clearly all day without them in.

HOW IS CORNEA ABRASION TREATED

You must seek immediate medical attention at the ER or from an eye professional for the most serious corneal abrasions. If you experience any vision loss, eye pain, or bloodshot, teary eyes, get medical attention right away. During the healing process, refrain from rubbing your eye.

To avoid infection, you are typically given topical antibiotic eye drops. The recommended dosage is around 4 times per day for 7 days. Wearing contact lenses is not permitted while the wound is healing. The majority of corneal abrasions will usually heal in 24 to 48 hours. A cold patch and some rest are advised.

How is a corneal abrasion treated?

This question and the one before it are extremely similar. So, my response will be comparable.

The response is based on:

Does the abrasion appear to be healing, or has it been there for a while (a few days) and is not appearing to?

Was the abrasion "Clean" or was it brought on by a contaminated object or piece of plant matter?

shallow or deep? Is it perforated or not?

the center or the periphery

Is your eye health or not?

You see, the solutions change depending on the situation.

Lubricants, mainly ointments rather than drops, maybe NSAID drops for pain, and possibly bandaging contact lenses are short-term treatments (for clean, uncontaminated abrasions).

Antibiotic drops or cream (ointment is typically qHS); it's possible to debride and culture before administering antibiotics (perhaps contaminated abrasion).

Find out why the abrasion is not healing for long-term treatment. Infected? Could it be HSV keratitis and not an abrasion? brain-shaped cornea? Recurrent corneal erosion, inadequate lubrication, exposure, anesthetic usage, self-inflicted injury, etc.

We no longer advise "pressure patching" closed eyes for corneal abrasions, which brings up two crucial considerations. It hinders healing and raises the possibility of infection being undiagnosed.

Never, ever provide topicals to patients.
drops of anesthetic to manage the discomfort.

What Is The Treatment? To prevent an infection from occurring in your eye, your doctor may advise using antibiotic eye drops or ointment. Along with pain medication, they could also give you prescription eyedrops to reduce pain and redness. To prevent light from irritating your eye, they could tape it shut and ask you to wear a patch over it.

WHAT IS SIGNS POINTS TO A CORNEAL SCRATCHED

One of the most typical eye injuries is a corneal abrasion, often known as a scratched cornea or scratched eye. Significant discomfort, red eyes, weeping, hazy vision, and sensitivity to light are possible symptoms of a scratched cornea.

Any object that comes into contact with the eye's surface can erode the cornea. However, compared to situations that happen frequently and cause abrasions, a trauma like being poked in the eye is less likely to result in corneal abrasion.

Makeup brushes are a common source of corneal abrasions.

branches of trees

A pet Office clutter

Dune and sand

Wet Eye

incorrect contact lens usage

sporting goods

The likelihood of corneal abrasions might be increased by dry eyes and incorrect contact lens use. Due to the lack of moisture in the eye, people who have dry eyes at night may actually tear the corneal epithelium while opening their eyes. The possibility of a scratched cornea is further increased by damaged contact lenses or prolonged lens usage.

Even though it's a natural instinct, you shouldn't rub your eye when you feel like something is in it. Rubbing your eye could aggravate the abrasion. The best thing to do is to rinse your eye with a sterile saline eye wash or multipurpose contact solution because bacteria can be found in both tap and bottled water. Seek quick assistance from an eye care expert if pain, redness, or other discomfort persists.

Your eye will be examined by an optometrist or ophthalmologist using eye drops to numb it as they assess the severity of the abrasion. Your eye may be swabbed for an eye culture if an infection is suspected.

MEIBOMIAN GLAND DYSFUNCTION

Meibomian gland dysfunction (MGD) is a catch-all term for a variety of meibomian gland conditions, including congenital and acquired conditions. Changes in the content of the tear film as a result of disturbed meibomian gland activity have an adverse effect on the quality and amount of meibum produced, which in turn has an adverse influence on the health of the ocular surface. Following this, there may be an increase in tear evaporation, hyperosmolarity, inflammation, and ocular surface injury. This could result in discomfort, blurred vision, and a dry eye sensation. The pathophysiology, causes, and effects of MGD on the ocular surface are all covered in this review article, along with how it relates to dry eye.

The rate of gland secretion has historically been used to categorize MGD.

1 Meibomian gland blockage or hyposecretion (either cicatricial or non-cicatricial) are considered low delivery states, whereas meibomian gland hypersecretion is considered a high delivery condition. All of these conditions

are further divided into main and secondary causes; for instance, seborrheic dermatitis and acne rosacea are secondary causes of both obstructive non-cicatricial and hypersecretory MGD. Mucus membrane pemphigoid is a secondary cause of obstructive, cicatricial MGD.

Within these subcategories, a low delivery status marked by gland blockage is the most frequent mechanism for MGD. Epithelial hyperkeratinization, which causes duct obstruction, meibum stasis, cystic dilation, and eventually disuses acinar atrophy and gland dropout, is thought to represent the underlying pathogenesis. 3–5 Recent research has expanded on this paradigm and identifies aberrant meibocytes as a significant factor in MGD. 6,7 Pathophysiologic research examining the effects of intrinsic (such as age) and extrinsic (such as environmental stress) MGD risk factors on meibocyte development and renewal provide evidence for the function of the meibocyte in MGD.

Aging MGD is known to be a danger from aging. 8 Age-related shrinkage of the meibomian gland acinar epithelial cells results in decreased lipid synthesis9, changed meibum composition, and altered neutral and polar lipid profiles. 10 Aged meibomian glands have decreased meibocyte differentiation, decreased meibocyte cell renewal, decreased meibomian gland size, and increased inflammatory cell infiltration, as observed in human and mouse models. These changes are likely what causes these changes. Peroxisome proliferator-activated receptor gamma (PPAR) expression has been found to be downregulated in correlation with these alterations. Nuclear receptor protein PPAR controls lipid production and meibocyte differentiation, which helps to generate and maintain meibomian glands. The reduced meibocyte differentiation and lipid synthesis seen with age, which results in gland atrophy and a hyposecretory state, is assumed to be caused by PPAR down-regulation. It is interesting to note that in this mouse model of MGD, gland blockage and hyperkeratinization were not shown to be contributing factors.

Stress due to Environment Stress from the environment also contributes to MGD. In a mouse model, low humidity-induced desiccating stress specifically caused several meibocyte-related abnormalities, such as a 3-fold increase in basal acinar cell proliferation, a changed protein/lipid ratio in the meibum, and irregular meibocyte differentiation, and a reduction in meibocyte stem cells. Since the protein to lipid ratios drop as meibum moves from the acini to the central duct under normal circumstances, these are probably linked. But animals under desiccating stress did not show this drop, indicating that the enhanced cellular proliferation and turnover resulted in altered meibocyte activity and a failure to remove protein from the meibum. Enhanced meibum production can occur as a short-term side effect of increased proliferation, which can also cause ductal dilatation. Long-term meibocyte depletion can lead to gland atrophy and hyposecretion as the number of active meibocytes decreases. Additionally, a larger protein/lipid ratio makes meibum more viscous, which has a detrimental effect on the integrity of the tear film.

Stem Cell Replacement Together, our results indicate that the reduction of meibocyte stem cells is a long-term effect of aging and environmental stress. The loss of acinar meibocytes and meibomian gland dropout seen in MGD can result from stem cell exhaustion. There has been disagreement over the identity and placement of meibomian gland stem cells; some studies situate them along the central duct, while others locate them at the junction of the ductal and acinar basal cells. The latter position in the junction between ductal and acinar basal cells was supported by a recent article that looked at many animal models. Additionally, different stem cell origins for various meibomian gland components have been discovered. Acini started from a single stem cell, whereas ducts came from progenitor cells with a variety of origins.

It's interesting to note that a connection between stress and aging has also been found in the cornea. The amount of limbal epithelial stem cells and their capacity for regeneration are partially measured by the thickness of the corneal epithelium. The eye experiences numerous times of stress over the course of a lifetime, during which stem cells multiply and restore normal equilibrium. The number and proliferative ability of corneal epithelial stem cells decline with age, similar to meibomian glands, which is observed as a decrease in epithelial thickness.

The potential impact of MGD risk factors on meibocytes

It is now clear that other factors previously linked to MGD, such as hormones, systemic and topical drugs, nutrition, and the ocular microbiota, can also alter meibocytes as a result of the developing concept that meibocyte dysfunction underpins MGD. Meibomian glands can also be diminished, absent, or replaced in a number of congenital illnesses, as well as affected by external factors such as the use of contact lenses.

a hormonal nature Meibomian glands have androgen and estrogen receptors, and meibocytes have the enzymes required for the intracrine synthesis and metabolism of sex steroids. In general, androgens promote meibum production and reduce inflammation, whereas estrogens promote inflammation. Thousands of genes, including those involved in lipid dynamics and PPAR signaling, are regulated by androgens in the human meibomian glands. Clinical cases of MGD have been reported in a variety of androgen-depleted conditions, including those treated with anti-androgen medications for benign prostatic hypertrophy or prostate cancer, those with total androgen insensitivity syndrome, and those with Sjogren's syndrome. Changes in lipid profiles and meibomian gland production were seen in each of these situations.

Systems-wide Medications The meibomian glands severely atrophy after using 13-cis-retinoid acid (Accutane, Roche Pharmaceuticals, Switzerland). Retinoids reduced mature lipid-laden acinar cells, thickened the ductal epithelium, and reduced acinar tissue in hamster models. Retinoic acid binds to nuclear receptors, altering gene transcription, which reduces the amount of acinar tissue in meibomian glands and prevents the formation of lipid-rich meibomian acinar cells. These results have been clinically linked to meibum hyposecretion, which affects tear osmolality and evaporation and causes symptoms of dry eyes.

Medications for the Skin The function of the meibomian gland has been discovered to be altered by several topical medicines. Topical epinephrine usage resulted in hyperkeratinization of the duct epithelium, which produced meibomian gland dilatation and clogging. Meibomian gland morphology alterations, such as reduced acinar area, acinar density, and homogenous acinar wall morphology, are linked to glaucoma drugs (such as topical beta blockers, prostaglandin analogs, and carbonic anhydrase inhibitors).

Nutrient Intake The symptoms and indicators of dry eye, as well as the expressibility and quality of meibum in MGD, have all been observed to improve with the administration of oral fatty acids. Consuming omega-3 fatty acids is specifically linked to changes in the polar lipid profile and lower levels of saturated fatty acids in the secretions of the meibomian gland. Omega-3 supplements also reduce the inflammatory lipid mediator profile in tears and ocular surface inflammation (as determined by HLA-DR) in dry eye patients. Flaxseed oil, fish oil, and olive oil are a few examples of foods that could be a good source of omega-3 fatty acids. Additionally, since the PPAR pathway is downregulated in MGD as previously mentioned, it may be advantageous to therapeutically target this pathway using agonists such as pharmaceuticals (thiazolidinediones: pioglitazone, troglitazone, and rosiglitazone) or dietary supplements (conjugated linoleic acid [vegetables, fruits, nuts, grains, and seeds; linseed oil] or docosahex

The microbiome of the Ocular Surface The cholesterol esters in the meibum may encourage the growth of commensal organisms like Staphylococcus aureus on the border of the eyelid. By degrading neutral fats and esters and releasing glycerides and free fatty acids (polar lipids) into the tear film, these commensal bacteria change the composition of meibum. In the absence of an infection, this happens as a result of the release of bacterial products (such as toxins and lipases). The mucin layer becomes hydrophobic as a result of the polar lipids diffusing through the water into it. The tear film becomes unstable as a result. Moreover, hyperkeratinization may be impacted by the conversion of triglycerides into free fatty acids. Demodex mite infestation has also been linked to MGD; in one study, nearly half

(46.8%) of MGD patients had Demodex present. Demodex's role in MGD is unclear, nevertheless, as it is frequently present in human hair follicles as a whole.

Using Contact Lenses Contact lens wear is linked to diminished meibomian gland shape and function. Meibomian gland dropout is more common in contact lens wearers, and the changes appear permanent. Additionally, anomalies in the lid margin and meibum quality are positively connected with the frequency of contact lens wear. While the underlying pathophysiology is unknown, theories include mechanical damage disrupting the meibomian glands, clogging caused by an accumulation of desquamated epithelial cells at gland orifices, and/or chronic inflammation.

Congenital Diminishment Meibomian glands might be missing or less developed at birth. Turner syndrome, ectrodactyly with ectodermal dysplasia and cleft-lip and-palate (ECC syndrome), and anhidrotic ectodermal dysplastic syndrome all exhibit congenital absence of glands. 49 Stub-like rudiments may be mostly absent or may appear as yellow streaks on the tarsal conjunctival surface. The surviving glands are frequently longer and larger than before, with the proximal end folded into the horizontal meridian or hooked back in a hairpin shape. 50

Replacement from Birth When a person has distichiasis, their meibomian glands are all replaced with eyelashes. Due to eyelash misdirection, this results in meibum insufficiency as well as ocular surface damage. Distichiasis can develop as a side effect of either the autosomal dominant disorder lymphoedema or a metaplastic reaction in mucocutaneous disease of the lids.

TREATMENT FOR KERATOCONUS

Your eye doctor (ophthalmologist or optometrist) will examine your eyes and perform an eye exam in order to identify keratoconus. He or she might perform additional exams to get a better idea of your cornea's shape.

There are several tests to identify keratoconus.

Choices

retinal refraction In this test, your eye doctor measures your eyes using specialized equipment to look for visual issues. He or she might ask you to look through a phoropter, a device with wheels of various lenses, to determine which combination provides you with the clearest vision. To examine your eyes, some doctors may use a retinoscope, a hand-held device.

Slit-lamp analysis In this test, your doctor shines a vertical beam of light directly onto the surface of your eye while seeing it through a low-powered microscope. He or she assesses the curvature of your cornea and scans your eye for any further potential issues.

Keratometry. In order to identify the basic shape of your cornea, your eye doctor will direct a circle of light at it and measure the reflection.

digital corneal mapping. A precise shape map of your cornea is produced by special photographic examinations like corneal tomography and corneal topography. The thickness of your cornea can also be determined using corneal tomography. Early keratoconus symptoms can frequently be identified by corneal tomography before the disease is obvious under a slit lamp.

Treatment

The inflexibility of your keratoconus and how fleetly it's progressing will determine how you're treated. In general, there are two ways to treat keratoconus by reducing the complaint's progression and by enhancing your vision.

Corneal collagen cross-linking may be advised to decelerate or stop the progression of your keratoconus if it's formerly present. You might not bear a corneal transplant in the unborn thanks to this more recent procedure. still, neither keratoconus nor vision is bettered by thistreatment.The degree of keratoconus determines whether you can ameliorate your vision. Contact lenses or eyeglasses can be used to treat mild to moderate keratoconus. The liability of this being a long- term remedy increases if your cornea becomes stable over time or as a result of cross-linking. Some keratoconus cases witness advanced complaints- related corneal scarring or difficulty wearing contact lenses.

Surgery for corneal transplantation may be needed in these patients.Lenses either soft contact lenses or eyeglasses. In early keratoconus, hazy or malformed vision can be treated with spectacles or soft contact lenses. But when the shape of their corneas changes, people constantly need to alter their tradition for eyeglasses or contacts.brittle contact lenses. The coming step in treating more advanced keratoconus is constantly the use of hard(rigid, gas passable) contact lenses. Although wearing hard lenses can be painful at first, numerous individualities get used to it and they can offer excellent vision. Your corneas can be fitted with this kind of lens.supplementary lenses. Your croaker

can advise" piggybacking" a hard contact lens over a soft bone

if rigid lenses are uncomfortable.hybrid optics For further comfort, these contact lenses have a establishment center and a softer ring around the edge. mongrel lenses may be preferred by those who can not wear hard contact lenses.lense scleral. When you have advanced keratoconus, these lenses can help with veritably irregular shape changes in your cornea. Scleral lenses sit on the white element of the eye(sclera), not the cornea, and vault over the cornea without touching it, unlike conventional contact lenses which rest on the cornea.Make careful to have your rigid or scleral connections fitted by an eye croaker

with experience in treating keratoconus if you wear connections. Regular examinations are also needed to make sure the fitting is still applicable. Your cornea could be harmed by an uncomfortable lens.

Therapy Collagen Cross-linking in the cornea. In this fashion, eyedrops containing riboflavin are applied to the cornea, and it's also exposed to ultraviolet light. As a result, the cornea becomes cross-linked, harshening it to stop fresh shape changes. By stabilizing the cornea beforehand in the complaint, corneal collagen cross-linking may help to lessen the liability of progressive vision loss.the surgery you have severe corneal thinning, corneal scarring, poor vision indeed with the strongest corrective lenses, or difficulty using any form of contact lenses, surgery may be necessary. Surgical druthers

include the following, depending on the position of the bulging cone and the soberness of your condition keratoplasty with penetration. You'll presumably bear a cornea transplant if you have severe corneal thinning or scarring(keratoplasty). A full- cornea transplant is a penetration keratoplasty. The central cornea of your eye is fully removed during this treatment and replaced with patron tissue.Anterior deep lamellar keratoplasty(DALK). The DALK fashion protects the cornea's internal filling(endothelium).

By doing this, it's possible to help the rejection of this vital interior filling, which can be with a full- consistency transplant.The success rate of cornea transplants for keratoconus is typically relatively high, but graft rejection, blurred vision, infection, and presbyopia are all implicit side goods. After entering a corneal transplant, wearing hard contact lenses is generally more comfortable and is constantly used to treat astigmatism.

CORNEAL TRANSPLANT FROM GORMANDIZERS (PIG)

according to a recent study, implants made from gormandizer skin have given eyeless people their sightback.

The implant employed in the study is manufactured from gormandizer collagen protein and is a duplicate of the mortal cornea, which is the transparent portion of the eye that covers the iris and pupil and allows light to enter.In the airman trial, which was reported in the journal Nature Biotechnology, the implants helped 20 people with damaged or unhealthy corneas recapture their vision. Prior to the operation, 14 subjects were fullyblind.Patients from India and Iran suffered from keratoconus, a complaint in which the cornea gradation ally thins and protrudes outward.According to the study, all of the cases had better vision 24 months after getting the implants.The study's generators, a group of scientists from Sweden, India, and Iran, saw the implants as a implicit result for scarce mortal corneal transplants.According to experts, there are around 12.7 million people on the cornea transplant staying list, and there's only one cornea accessible for every 70 people who bear the transplant, according to the study.Poorer to middle-income nations in Asia, Africa, and the Middle East have indeed less access to bestowed corneas.

www.ingramcontent.com/pod-product-compliance
Lightning Source LLC
LaVergne TN
LVHW052112160826
845678LV00015B/3513

* 9 7 9 8 8 4 6 8 1 9 6 3 4 *